Where Did I Put My Map?

A Little Manual for Caregivers of Alzheimer's Patients

by

Jude Gann R.N.

authorHOUSE

1663 LIBERTY DRIVE, SUITE 200
BLOOMINGTON, INDIANA 47403
(800) 839-8640
www.authorhouse.com

First published by AuthorHouse 06/08/04

ISBN: 1-4184-1848-X (e)
ISBN: 1-4184-1849-8 (sc)

Library of Congress Control Number: 2004105305

Printed in the United States of America
Bloomington, Indiana

This book is printed on acid-free paper.

Table of Contents

FORWARD

This little manual has been a work-in-progress. It began as my personal resource list and information file. As it grew, I realized that many other people were in the same circumstance as I was. So, I began to collect and organize my information. This is the result, I hope this will be helpful to you in your journey.

The first thing I want to say to you who are reading this is: "Your life is forever changed!" The best thing to do now is to face it directly and prepare adequately for what is to come. There is nothing easy about dealing with Alzheimer's disease. You can make a choice to walk the pathway that God has placed before you with joy and humor and look for the good in every situation, or to become overwhelmed, depressed, and saddened to such an extent that you may become the patient yourself. Statistically, caregivers often die before the patient. Don't let yourself become a part of that statistic.

The second thing is that I will pray for you. I have personally walked this road and could not have come to this place without the persistent prayers of folk who loved and cared for me. God is faithful! No matter how difficult your road may become, He will walk it with you. Your loved one is in a special place of care in the hands of God, and is generally not aware that his life has become tragic. Try to see the humor in the things that will happen, and share your laughter with your loved one. Learn to put the past in the past, take one thing at a time, prioritize your life to accommodate your present task, and remember Who it is that walks beside you.

Lastly, I dedicate whatever comes of this little manual to my sweet, loving husband, H.B. Gann, who passed away on May 31, 2001. Without him my life would have been very different and very bland. I was blessed to be a part of his journey and I am grateful for the sweet years of partnership we had together.

Jude Gann, RN
2001

INTRODUCTION

I cannot even envision the magnitude of the number of families that are trying to cope with someone with Alzheimer's disease, or with some other form of dementia that interferes with daily living. As our population in the United States grows, and as medical technology allows for longer lives, the population over age 65 grows exponentially. This group of folk has been called the "Baby Boomers." I, myself, belong to this group. We have been privileged to live in a time when our country was prosperous and our lives were blessed with good health and comfortable surroundings. Advances in medicine have allowed us to extend our lives and to live reasonably well with diseases that previously would have been fatal early in our lives. All of these wonderful medical advances have come with a price.

According to statistics issued by the Administration on Aging, the number of people with limitations to their activities of daily living (ADL) in 1990 was 18.8%. By the year 2040 this number will grow to 21.4%. Already there are too few facilities available for long term care. Even if we began today on a massive building program, we could not provide enough beds quickly enough to meet the need for services that will be demanded in the coming years. In addition to the shortage of facilities, there is now a large shortage of nurses. Even acute care hospitals are scrambling to provide adequate nursing care for their patients. Nursing schools are recruiting students, but cannot keep up with the demand.

Further, in addition to the shortage of nurses, there is a huge shortage of professional home-care providers. People who opt to keep their loved ones at home instead of an institution find that help is scarce and expensive.

This group of "Baby Boomers" has also come to rely upon our government to pay for their medical care, as well as the cost of long term care institutions. The expense of inpatient care has skyrocketed, and many must pay out-of-pocket to the tune of thousands of dollars each month. Outpatient care is an attractive option financially, however difficult it is to arrange and maintain in our very busy lifestyles.

The result is that there is an increasing need for training and support services for family or spouse caregivers. Those who have chosen, or been financially forced, to go this route are largely left to their own devices to discover how to be a good caregiver, and stay alive and healthy themselves.

This manual is intended to be a step-by-step tool for at-home caregivers. I have tried to incorporate most of the important or daily issues; however, I may have omitted something with which you are struggling. If so, I am sorry. Do not struggle alone. Find help, if not here, the bookstore, the internet, the counselors at long term care facilities, friends, family, support groups...keep looking!!

CHAPTER 1:

OVERVIEW

WHAT YOU NEED TO KNOW ABOUT ALZHEIMER'S DISEASE:

1) What is it?
    Alzheimer's Disease is an age-related progressive disorder of the central nervous system, characterized by chronic cognitive dysfunction. It is the most prevalent of all nonreversible dementias. Alzheimer's Disease rarely develops before age 40, and usually begins after the age of 65. It is slightly more common in women than in men, and afflicts between 3 and 5 million individuals in the United States.

2) What causes it?
    The exact cause of Alzheimer's Disease remains unknown; however, there may be one or more faulty genes responsible for its development. It is believed that the buildup of amyloid placque, the development of neurofibrillary tangles, and changes in neurons contribute to the progressive loss of function seen in Alzheimer's Disease. It has been shown to have a genetic link.

3) How is it diagnosed?
    Alzheimer's Disease is difficult to diagnose, especially in the early stages where it resembles many other disorders. It cannot be definitively diagnosed in a living person. The diagnosis is usually made by a clinical examination including a medical history, a physical examination, neuropsychological tests, and other tests of the person's mental ability. Often a CT scan, an MRI, an MRS, or a PET scan may be used to detect abnormalities in the brain.

4) What are the signs, symptoms, and stages?
    The most definitive signs are the "Four A's:"
    a) Amnesia is the inability to learn new information or to recall previously learned information.
    b) Agnosia is the failure to recognize or identify objects despite intact sensory function.
    c) Aphasia is a language disturbance that can manifest in both understanding and expression of the spoken word.
    d) Apraxia is the inability to carry out motor activities despite intact motor function.

5) WHAT ARE THE STAGES OF ALZHEIMER'S DISEASE?

    STAGE ONE: - EARLY CONFUSION
            Forgetfulness is beginning to interfere with daily routine
            Difficulty concentrating
            Difficulty learning new material
            Good days outnumber the bad days
            Loss of empathy for others

STAGE TWO: - LATE CONFUSION
>   Gets lost easily in unfamiliar places
>   Recent memory shows decline
>   Forgets appointments (doctors, dentists, hair-dresser, etc.)
>   Losing interest in world or community events
>   Beginning to have difficulty shopping
>   May refuse to admit anything is different
>   Covers behavior by accusing others – especially in the family

STAGE THREE: - EARLY DEMENTIA
>   Good days are less frequent
>   Confusion causes person to eat too much or too little food
>   Forgets names of grandchildren and friends
>   More easily frustrated
>   Difficulty following sequenced tasks, such as cooking a meal
>   Frequent repetition of particular subjects or stories
>   Has trouble finding words
>   May wander

STAGE FOUR: - MIDDLE DEMENTIA
>   Can no longer be alone, needs supervision
>   Difficulty with bathing; cannot accomplish bath alone or refuses
>   In the middle of a task asks, "What are we doing?"
>   Easily distracted
>   Made anxious if too many things are happening at once
>   Outbursts of fear, anger, and frustration
>   Sleep patterns change – may mix nights and days
>   Follows caregiver around constantly

STAGE FIVE: - LATE MIDDLE DEMENTIA
>   Need assistance in everything they do
>   Words no longer identified with their meaning
>   Difficulty in walking, rising from a chair, and standing
>   Poor judgement in where to put body parts as in sitting
>   Incontinence of urine and sometimes stool
>   Language becomes more incomprehensible

STAGE SIX: - PROFOUND DEMENTIA
>   Person must be fed
>   Incontinent
>   Communicates nonverbally all the time
>   Susceptible to pneumonia and complications as a result of
>   immobility

TERMINAL PHASE:
>   Person is bed-bound and requires constant care
>   Emaciated and helpless
>   The most frequent cause of death is pneumonia and other
>   infections with malnutrition and dehydration as contributing factors

CHAPTER 2:

HOME EVALUATION:

INSIDE YOUR HOME

GENERAL:

First, give careful consideration to the level of dementia experienced by your loved one. Plan accordingly, but allow for progressive changes. You may think you do not need to implement all of the suggestions listed below. Keep these things in mind, however, for a future day. Things may change unexpectedly, if you are prepared ahead of time the adjustment will be easier.

1)   DOORS AND GATES:
Install a <u>keyed</u> deadbolt lock on your front door. One of the most common problems associated with Alzheimer's is wandering. You will save yourself a lot of heartache if you do everything possible to prevent wandering outside of your home. You can purchase a plastic wrist-band keychain that you can wear on your arm at all times for convenience.

You may wish to install "baby-gates" in certain doorways or at the top or bottom of stairs, and place a padlock on them. Add this key to your wrist keychain for your convenience. You also may decide to shut or lock other inside doors as may be necessary.

2)   FALL PREVENTION:
Remove any throw rugs and keep floors clear of loose items. Clear all pathways through the home. Remove any extension cords as necessary.

3)   HOUSEHOLD ITEMS:
Put away or lock up any sharps, chemicals, and medications. If necessary, you can purchase a locked cabinet for needed medications. You can keep this key on your wrist keychain as well.

You may want to disconnect the toaster, disable your stove, and put childproof latches on cabinets and drawers wherever necessary. You can easily install cover plates on electric outlets for additional safety.

If you are financially able, you may want to consider installing motion activated lights in hallways and bathrooms for use at nighttime; installing an in-home video camera or closed circuit TV system; or even consider options for remodeling or for new building.

It is important to remove or paint over any "busy" wallpaper, and choose neutral solid colors for your walls. Busy wallpaper can be a great distraction to your patient and may be a large factor in constant and daily confusion.
Keep a complete list of emergency phone numbers near your telephone.
More information concerning this item is provided in the chapter on safety.

Television viewing and/or video movies will have to be monitored.

You should avoid viewing violent or noisy television or music.

People with dementia often cannot differentiate between people on the television screen and real people in the room. They may become overly agitated or frightened by some television content.

Providing a daily ritual and structure in your lifestyle will be very important.

Changes of any kind will cause anxiety and may lead to a "catastrophic reaction." Try to keep life simple if possible and avoid large numbers of people in the room at the same time.

> A "catastrophic reaction" is an overreaction to an event or stimulus in the form of anger, fear, anxiety, grief, or some other powerful emotion. It usually happens because the person does not understand what is going on, or the caregiver intervenes too roughly or too quickly. Never confront, always persuade. Never give orders, always make suggestions. Never push or pull roughly, always guide gently. If you show violence, you will receive violence. The best way to deal with it is to remove the cause.
>
> Remain calm, reassuring, patient.

BATHROOMS:

1) You can place a brightly colored sign on the bathroom door to identify it. A person who cannot find the bathroom, or remember where it is, will likely use inappropriate places in frustration.

2) Install grab-bars in necessary places such as the shower, beside the toilet, etc.

3) Remove locks on bathroom doors, especially ones that can be locked from the inside. Remove or lock up any medications.

4) Keep your water temperature BELOW 120 degrees to prevent scalding burns.

5) Elevate toilet seats and provide "arms" on toilets as necessary for stability.

6) Install large, easily turned faucet handles which are clearly marked, "Hot" and "Cold."

7) Install a hand-held shower extension to facilitate showering activities.

8) Install non-slip strips in tubs and showers.

9) Avoid using oils with bath or shower to prevent slipping and falling.

10) Be prepared to clean up unexpected messes in the bathroom, especially around the toilet area, without anger or blaming. Accidents will be a part of your life now.

KITCHEN:

The kitchen can be a dangerous place for a person with dementia.

Rearranging this area can be stressful for you and you may have to learn some new habits; but that will be less stressful than an injury or worse to your loved one.

1) Put away all of your breakable dishes and glassware. Avail yourself of the many new and wonderful plastic items and use disposables whenever possible.

2) Remove extension cords, cover electric outlets, and put away small household appliances such as toasters, mixers, blenders, etc.

3) You can disable your stove by removing the handles, or, if necessary, even turning off the gas completely.

4) Go through your silverware and knife drawer and remove all knives and other sharp instruments. Place them in a locked cabinet for now.

5) Go through your cupboards and put away or lock up any dangerous chemicals such as household bleach, ammonia, plant fertilizer, etc.

6) Put away or lock up all medications, even over-the-counter items such As vitamins, aspirin, cold remedies. Your loved one may easily mistake one item for another or not remember having taken a dose and take another, or none at all.

7) See the notes on Nutritional needs later in this book and stock your cupboards or pantry accordingly.

All of this probably seems overwhelming to you right now. However, the sooner you address these issues and learn to live differently, the more likely you are to have a less stressful outcome. Do not let yourself be lulled into thinking that your case does not require these things to be done. This is an instance where the old adage proves true: "An ounce of prevention is worth a pound of cure!"

SAFE ROOM FOR YOUR PATIENT:

If you have the room in your house it might be a helpful idea to create a "safe-room" for your patient. Try to find a room with easily cleaned floors such as linoleum; soft furniture with no sharp corners; a comfy chair; some favorite pictures; where you could even install a lock on the door; and dedicate this room to your loved one.

You may want to include in this room:
A large calendar
A clock with large numbers
A good light
A table for games or hobbies
A television or stereo
Some favorite music, videos, magazines, toys, puzzles, games, coloring or drawing items, or other hobby items that are personalized to your patient.

You may also want to provide a large box or basket of mismatched socks or towels and washcloths that can be folded and refolded.

If this room is not adjacent to a bathroom, you may also want to provide a bedside commode.

> One of the most treasured items will be a "Memory Book." This will
> include a collection of photos from your patient's childhood, marriage,
> travels, hobbies, grandchildren, etc. You can personalize it as necessary.
> You may even want to have the pages photocopied and bound in another
> book so your patient can carry it with him and you will not lose the
> original. This will be a loved and treasured item.

SAFE ROOM FOR THE CAREGIVER:

Another option would be a special room for the caregiver where you can go to find some comfort and quiet. You may even want to install a lock on the door. Certainly you will want to personalize this room as you wish. Do not feel guilty about secluding yourself here when things become overwhelming; and they WILL!

OUTSIDE YOUR HOME:

FENCES:

If you do not already have an adequate fence around your back yard, this is a necessity to which you will want to give serious consideration.
A strong fence with keyed padlocks on any gates will provide a safe place for your patient to be outside in appropriate weather, and will prevent your patient from wandering off unnoticed.

OUTBUILDINGS:

If you have any outbuildings in your yard, you may want to install locks on the doors. If you prefer, you can simply remove any dangerous items or substances that may be stored inside the building, and clean it out.
Be prepared to clean up if your patient thinks your outbuilding is an "outhouse!" Do not blame or scold if this should happen.

YARD SAFETY:

Be certain that there are not things in your yard that could be dangerous.
Not only should it be cleared of sharp stones or yard-tools, but poisonous plants should be removed or placed in some other area unreachable by your patient.

If you do not know which plants may be poisonous, you can call any Nursery or your local Extension Service for further information.

CHAPTER 3:

VEHICLE SAFETY

DRIVING:

In our country driving is a big part of everyday life and we vigorously defend our rights to have this freedom and control of our lives. Despite any resistance, families must address the problems surrounding their loved one's driving opportunities. Even early on this person is vulnerable to situations requiring quick decisions because his reaction time is impaired and his problem-solving abilities are easily overwhelmed. Removal of driving responsibilities eliminates the possibility of an unfortunate accident.

If your patient is unwilling to stop driving willingly enlist the help of his physician, attorney, insurance agent, mental health professional, or trusted friend. The physician may be willing to write on a prescription blank "No Driving Privileges." This will serve as a reminder to the person, and a tool for family members and/or law enforcement personnel. You may want to remove keys or dismantle the car's starter if necessary. Understand the person's anger and resentment, but avoid confrontations and stand your ground. This decision can be a matter of life and death.

CHILDPROOF LOCKS:

Most vehicles today are equipped with child-proof locks on the back doors. These are valuable tools when your patient is in your vehicle.

It goes without saying that seat-belts should ALWAYS be worn correctly. It will be safer for everyone if your patient is seated in the back seat of your vehicle, seat belt attached, and child-proof locks in order. Some patients may become so agitated, they may distract the driver unnecessarily, or they may even attempt to exit the vehicle while it is in motion if they are not properly restrained.

Convincing your patient to enter or exit the vehicle may become a problem. Patience and ingenuity will decide the outcome. Distraction techniques can be learned and employed as necessary.

CHAPTER 4:

NUTRITION

You will want to learn all you can about basic food information and about the food-guide pyramid. Nutrition will become a big issue, so prepare in advance with information. Many excellent books are available concerning nutrition and helpful tips can be obtained from the internet or from friends at your support group.

Give up the idea of "three meals per day." You will have better success with six or eight small meals or with a constant supply of high calorie, nutrient dense, finger-foods. If your patient is a diabetic you will need to adjust these foods to accommodate the limitations. Make a list of your patient's favorite foods, both for your own reference and for any outside caregivers who may become involved. You may wish to consult a dietitian if you have unanswered questions.

Bottled water is a life-saver. It is easily available, easy to handle, and good for your patient. Supplement drinks, like Ensure, are a must. You may want to consult your physician as to which specific one would be best for your patient. They come in many varieties and flavors and can be purchased at your local grocery store.

You may want to create a new recipe book including all of your new ideas for favorite and nutritionally sound finger-foods and appropriate meals. This will not only be a useful tool in your kitchen, but will be a fun hobby for you in the process.

Learn to use a blender whenever necessary. Many ordinary foods can be easily pureed for easier eating –they will taste the same. You can puree hot-dogs, catchup and bun and all; beef stew, any meats; vegetables, etc. Use your imagination. Your Alzheimer's patient will soon "forget" how to eat, so be creative to facilitate nutritional needs.

Be prepared for stress and mess. Never get in a hurry – these patients react very poorly to being rushed. Use a "sippy-cup"; a towel with a tie-on for a bib; and plastic utensils. Sitting down for a meal at a table is not usually workable, but keep up your previous routines as long as possible.

CHAPTER 5:

HEALTH CARE INFORMATION, DRUGS, TREATMENTS

Make a list of all prescription drugs with all information and instructions. An example of such a list follows. You may prefer to create your own. Be certain to include all "over-the counter" items as well, such as Aspirin, Vitamins, herbal remedies, etc.

Keep copies of all health information as well as copies of all physician records and hospital records on file. They can be stored in expandable file folders, or even kept in a 3-ring binder by date or location. Use your own method, but keep them!

A sample health-information card with a picture of your patient is included here. This may be filled out completely (changed as often as is necessary) and, importantly, will contain a photo. This information should be kept in your wallet or purse. It will be asked of you by every physician or health care institution where you go, and you will be going more frequently than you wish.

Adapt a Medical Administration Record (MAR) to keep careful track of all medications administered by dose, strength, time of day and person administering. This will prevent any potential medication over-doses or under-doses, and will relieve your mind about appropriate medications. If you wish to obtain further information concerning drugs you may find what you need on the internet or in one of the many excellent drug books available at your local bookstore. It is wise to know what medications you are giving and why, as well as what they may do to your patient. Ask your primary care physician to go over the list carefully and eliminate what is not necessary.

Purchase a good pillcrusher, medicine cups, dose-packed medications when available, and a daily or weekly pill holder for your convenience. Consult your pharmacist about which medications may be available in liquid form because your patient may be unable or unwilling to swallow pills. Also be certain you know which pills may be safely crushed and put into a spoon of ice-cream or applesauce. Some medications may not or cannot be crushed.

Your physician and your pharmacist are valuable resources. They can help you to monitor medications, and problems with medications, and help you adjust medications as necessary. They will know which medications react differently in elderly persons, or persons with kidney disease. Even a simple thing such as a Tylenol for a headache can produce a terrible result if given to a person with certain medical problems. I cannot stress too strongly the need to keep in close communication with physicians and pharmacists, and to make certain the primary care physician is fully aware of ALL medications given to your patient by any and every specialist or other physician you may be seeing.

CHAPTER 6:

PERSONAL CARE

It is very important to obtain proper identification for your loved one in case they should become lost or wander off somewhere. An attractive metal ID bracelet can be purchased at any jewelry store which includes the person's name on the front and a notation on the underside such as "Memory Impaired," as well as a phone number. This bracelet should be placed on the arm with the latch removed and the chain permanently hooked together so it cannot easily be taken off. It can be worn at all times, even in the tub or shower without problem.

A wide variety of alarms are available for your use. A bed-alarm or chair alarm that sounds when the person attempts to get up, and a door-alarm that sounds if the door is opened would be most helpful.

If your patient is prone to falls, a bicycle helmet is useful to prevent head injuries. Shoes should be properly fitted, sturdy, and have velcro fasteners. Pull-up diapers are now available for minor accidents if your patient is still mobile. Later, you may want to switch to tab-fastener diapers for your convenience.

When you are out in public, such as walking in the mall or the park, you can utilize a set of child's mitten clips. These clips may be attached, one to the sleeve of your patient and the other to your sleeve. This will allow for some freedom, but will let you know if they turn to wander off elsewhere.

It is best not to offer choices. Too many choices will be confusing to the patient and will be frustrating to you when they cannot make a decision.

> You pick the clothing to be worn and offer it one item at a time.
> You pick the foods to be eaten.
> You pick everything, and simply offer it to the patient one thing at a time.
> Keep your sentences short and simple. Complicated sentences are not understood.
> Do not "talk down" to your patient. They are not children even though they may act as such. Consider how you would like to be addressed if it were you in this circumstance.

BATH TIME:

Bath time can become one of the biggest issues with which you will have to deal. Persons with Alzheimer's are literally afraid of water. They don't know what it is and they don't like the feel of it on their skin. Don't force bathing. Look for opportunities, and learn distraction techniques. It is not necessary to have a bath every day as long as reasonable care is taken to clean up where necessary. A "sponge-bath" may prove easier to manage than trying to convince someone to climb into a bathtub or a shower. If necessary, ask for help from someone else in the family or from a professional home care person for bathing. Incontinence will increase. Be prepared to deal with it quietly and carefully.

CLOTHING NEEDS

Getting ourselves dressed is a daily activity we generally take for granted. However, persons with cognitive disabilities will have problems with this simple task that can lead to great frustration, misunderstanding, and catastrophic reactions.

Avoid buttons and zippers whenever possible. Substitute velcro closures.

Use easy, comfortable, warm clothing. Sweat shirts and pants are a wonderful invention and the shirts may be split up the front or back and velcro sewn in to make it easier to put on and take off. If you are able to sew, it is easy to do yourself. If not, you can find a seamstress who will be willing to do this simple task for you.

Don't offer choices, you pick the clothing to be worn. Offer it one piece at a time and allow sufficient time for it to be put on – hurrying is NOT an option. Some patients will want to put on several pair of pants or shirts, or may take clothing from other family members and try to wear it. Do not become angry or forceful if this happens, and if weather permits simply leave them in their layered or mismatched outfits. It isn't worth getting upset over clothing choices.

EXERCISE AND ACTIVITY

The ability to move body parts independently is a function most people take for granted. Mobility or lack of it has a significant impact on an individual's physiological, psychosocial, and developmental well-being. When there is an alteration in mobility, many body systems are at risk for impairment. Impaired mobility may result in decreased joint range of motion, loss of muscular strength and endurance, loss of bone mass and strength, cardiovascular deterioration, respiratory problems, metabolic imbalances, pressure ulcers, and decreased urinary function. Daily exercise is critical to a continued physical well-being. Walking is the easiest to do, and when weather prevents a walk around the block, a walk around the living room several times will do nicely. Video tapes are available to assist you with different levels of daily exercising. Even a bed-bound person needs a certain amount of daily exercise. You may consult a physical therapist or activity director for assistance tailored to your needs.

DEALING WITH PROBLEMS:

BODY FUNCTIONS:

It is important to remember that body functions are a normal and natural part of being alive. Persons with dementia may not remember how to deal with these daily functions. It can be frustrating and embarrassing, both for the patient and for the caregiver. You will have to put on your best patience and treat this person as you would like to be treated were it you in this position.

PERI-CARE:

Good hygiene is vital. Deposits of urine and fecal matter can cause infections, pressure sores, and odors. The area must be washed thoroughly each time. A spray-on preparation is available for this purpose. Baby-wipes are an easy-to-use alternative. Applying a soothing powder or ointment and changing clothing and pads frequently will make this job easier.

<u>INCONTINENCE:</u>

Incontinence is common in people with dementia. People often forget when they last used the bathroom; they may not be able to remember where the bathroom is located, or how to use the toilet when they get there; or they may not be able to identify the feelings that signal us when to go. Although incontinence may be temporary early in the disease, it will become a permanent problem as time passes. Some helpful things you can do are:

Tape a picture of a toilet on the bathroom door, and leave lights on at night for easier access.

Utilize clothing that is easy to remove, without buttons and zippers.

Establish a routine for toileting. Cue your patient every two hours or so, and limit the amounts of liquid intake in the evenings.

Note behaviors that may signal the need to go. This may include restlessness, clutching at the groin area, pacing, or facial expressions of discomfort or pain.

Absorbent pads or diapers may be worn. You will find a wide variety of these available at your local drugstore or grocery. Try different types to ascertain which will work best for your situation. Be sure to change them often.

Place a waterproof cover over your mattress and be prepared to change the bed linens often.

Avoid beverages with a diuretic effect, such as coffee, tea, grapefruit juice, and colas.

Do not berate the person when accidents happen. Make it a habit to check often and clean up without recriminations. It is YOU who will have to make adjustments, your loved one is no longer able to deal with this as before. It is a mistake to think that you can "retrain" this person concerning toileting.

CHAPTER 7:

BASIC NURSING SKILLS

It will be important for you to obtain instruction on some simple and basic nursing skills. Perhaps you are acquainted with a nurse who will assist you to learn. If not, a home-health agency can provide someone to teach you what you will need to know. From the following list you may choose to add or delete items to suite your situation:

HAND WASHING:

The most important and most basic technique in preventing and controlling transmission of infection is hand washing. Routine hand washing may be performed with soap in any convenient form. However, liquid soap is more convenient and less likely to harbor microorganisms.

BED MAKING:

I know it is a pain in the neck to change bed linens several times each day. Residual body fluids will not only cause unwanted odors, but may cause skin breakdown or infection. Resign yourself to becoming best friends with your washing machine.

TRANSFERRING:

With loss of coordination, moving from chair to bed or wheelchair, or even walking to the bathroom may become a difficult task. A physical therapist will be happy to give you some specialized instruction when needed. JUST ASK!!

SKIN CARE:

Prevention of decubitus ulcers and pressure sores is extremely important. This will become more of an issue as the disease progresses. It is critical to move a bed-bound patient every couple of hours to prevent skin breakdown.

WHEELCHAIR SAFETY:

If your patient uses a wheelchair, you will want to obtain some careful instruction about transferring in and out of it. Be certain that wheels are locked in place and foot and leg rests are out of the way. Talk with a physical therapist about which type will work for you, and check with your insurance company to see which type will be covered.

SHAVING:

It is not wise to use razors with blades that may cause cuts or infections. Purchase an electric razor, and keep it away from water sources.

NAIL AND FOOT CARE:

Feet and nails require special care to prevent infection, odors, and injury to soft tissues. Consult with a Podiatrist if necessary and ask for some instruction on cutting and cleaning.

TEMPERATURE, BLOOD PRESSURE, PULSE:

Inexpensive blood pressure cuffs may be purchased at your local drugstore. Instruction on how to use them may be obtained either from your pharmacist or your doctor's office. Having these items in your home will prevent many unnecessary trips to the doctor's office.

MEASURING INTAKE AND OUTPUT:

You may want to create a daily chart for measuring intake and output. Patients with dementia may forget to drink enough fluids and become dehydrated. Encouraging liquids will help prevent both urinary tract infections and constipation.

BODY MECHANICS:

It is important for you to use good body mechanics when handling your loved one. It will become more important as the disease progresses and he requires more and more assistance with daily tasks and with movement. If one is available, you may want to actually take a class in good body mechanics.

BREATHING TECHNIQUES:

Focusing on breathing will become an important tool for you as your frustration level increases. Stop what you are doing, breath in slowly through your nose to the count of four, using your belly instead of your chest for inspiration; hold this breath to the count of five; exhale slowly through pursed lips. You can do this as often as is necessary to help you cope. Remember: "Smell a rose, and blow out a candle."

BATHING:

We have discussed bathing elsewhere here. If you keep the perineal area clean and dry a daily bath is not always necessary. Sponge baths may be easier to accomplish than getting a bathtub or a shower. Persons with Alzheimer's disease become afraid of water. Do not force this issue. Arrange for help when you need it.

MOUTH CARE:

Daily mouth care is important. Getting dentures out of the mouth of a person with dementia may be difficult, but they should be cleansed daily. You will have to get very creative to make this happen. Sponge-swabs are a handy tool for mouth care as it is important to prevent thrush. If the mouth becomes sore or if thrush appears, ask your physician for some kind of "Swish and Swallow" preparation to use.

IMMOBILITY:

Amazingly, the human body needs daily activity. Even just walking around your living-room or back yard several times each day will help with mobility. Just be certain to remove items that may cause tripping or falling, and to allow for rest periods whenever necessary

HEARING IMPAIRED:

Many elderly persons are hearing impaired and make use of a variety of hearing aids. Since your patient will probably not remember, it will fall to you to take care of any aids. Remove the hearing aid at bedtime and displace the battery to preserve it. Check with your local hearing aid vendor regarding regular cleaning and care. Replace batteries whenever necessary and discard them properly. They are usually small and can be easily dropped or swallowed.

DISTRACTION TECHNIQUES:

Persons with dementia do not respond favorably to command-voice. If you confront them aggressively they will become more upset and may progress to a full-blown catastrophic reaction. Do whatever is necessary to learn distraction techniques, it will save you a lot of heartache. Speak softly and calmly, do not raise your voice. Ask about favorite activities or grandchildren. Gently stroke an arm, but do not reach for the forehead. They may think you are about to strike them and become more agitated. Never make sudden, unexpected movements toward their face or head. If necessary, stop what you are doing and sit down with them for a few minutes. Nothing is so important that it should cause conflict or fear.

DISTORTED THINKING:

People who must contend daily with the stress, anxiety, and frustrations of Alzheimer's caregiving often feel alone and afraid. It is important to take care of yourself and not allow distorted thinking to control your life. Help is readily available on the Internet or at your local bookstore about how to untwist your thinking. Please make every effort to become aware of what and how you are thinking and take steps to prevent problems and plan corrective actions. Knowledge is power!

THE 10 MOST COMMON FORMS OF DISTORTED THINKING:

1)   All Or Nothing: Don't allow yourself to think that one mistake makes you a total failure.
2)   Labeling: Making a mistake now and then does not make you a worthless person.
3)   Overgeneralization: Watch out for words like "always" or "never," such as "I always mess up.
4)   Mental Filtering: Complicated situations that involve both positive and negative elements may lead you to dwell on the negative.
5)   Discounting the Positive: "That doesn't count," or "that wasn't good enough."
6)   Jumping to Conclusions: Assuming the worst based on the evidence.
7)   Magnification: Exaggerating the importance of problems, shortcomings, and minor annoyances.
8)   Emotional Reasoning: Mistaking your emotions for reality.

9) "Should" and "Shouldn't" Statements: Other self-demanding words include "must," "ought to," and "have to." Go easy on yourself.

10) Personalizing the Blame: Taking responsibility for things beyond your control.

CHAPTER 8:

THE COGNITIVELY IMPAIRED PERSON IN AN ACUTE-CARE SETTING:

Persons with cognitive disorders require a milieu in which they are neither overstimulated nor understimulated. They have a right to a safe environment; free from injury, stress, and anxiety; free from misleading and frightening stimuli. Consideration should be given to the impact on these persons from such things as television, public address systems, pictures of animals or people on walls, and "busy" wallpapers. There is always a variety of persons who enter the room, bustling and hustling to get a particular job done in a hurry and leave again, often without even introducing themselves or explaining what they are about to do. Impaired persons need a warm, caring atmosphere where they can develop a trusting interpersonal relationship with their caregivers. They do better with a predictable routine, followed daily; and with close supervision. The very things most needed by these people is, in fact, the most difficult to provide in a busy, acute-care setting. The following is a short, alphabetic resource of information for your patient with a cognitive impairment:

ACTIVITIES: It is unrealistic to expect these patients to learn new skills.
Even small amounts of excitement can upset them. Look for ways to simplify activities.

APPROACHING: Approach these patients slowly. Explain what you are doing.
Approach from the side if at all possible; a direct approach in the face may frighten them.

BATHING: Many cognitively impaired persons have a great fear of water. Do not force this issue. A daily bath may not be necessary. You can sponge off necessary areas and quit.

COMMUNICATION: This is a key issue. Use short, simple sentences, but do not talk down to them. Communicate ONE thing at a time and wait for their response. NOT: "Now sit up and get dressed and eat your breakfast." Two or three requests may cause them to do nothing at all.

DEMANDS: Demands may come from loneliness, loss, being frightened.
Try to reassure the patient; be friendly; distract.

DISTRACTION: These patients are easily distracted by noise, people, television. If you want his attention, reduce the distractions.
Reminisce, ask about family members, be prepared to repeat and repeat.

EVALUATE: Needs and moods will change rapidly. Re-evaluate often.

FALLS: This person's gait may be unsteady. He may look alright one moment and fall the next. This is because he may "forget" how to walk.

GROOMING: Help and encourage the patient to do for himself as much as is possible. Praise and encouragement are important to help this person feel good when such tasks have become too much for him.

HOARDING: Hoarding, hiding, losing things are common. If something is misplaced please remember NOT to ask the patient where he put it...he will not remember. If this person wants to collect odd things, it is best to let her. "Cleaning out" her stash may prompt a suspicious reaction.

INAPPROPRIATE SEXUAL BEHAVIOR: Do not overreact! Distract with something else. The person is only doing what feels good.
Gently redirect his actions.

JERKING: Jerking (Myoclonus) and Tremors may be expected in a dementing illness. This may be due to drugs, ask your physician to evaluate medications as necessary. Do not command your patient to "Hold still!" They cannot.

JUDGEMENT: Judgement is impaired in this patient due to the dementing illness. The need to intervene increases with the potential risk to the patient.

KNOWLEDGE DEFICIT: Teaching or explanations may be difficult. You will have to repeat many times and then never be sure you were understood.

LEARNING: Memory, especially short-term memory, is key to learning.
This patient will generally be unable to learn new information. This will affect many areas. Logic cannot be processed; instruction may be difficult.

MEDICATIONS: Many medications contribute to confusion, especially in the elderly who may have more sensitivity. Administering medications may become difficult. These patients cannot follow instructions or learn new information. They may actually "forget" how to swallow. Their medications may need to be crushed and put in food or given in liquid form.
They may hoard or hide medications. Watch carefully, check in their mouth. You may find pills in the bedclothes or on the floor. Be very careful here.

MISINTERPRETATION: This may be due to vision or hearing problems.
It may be due to lighting or shadows.
Give factual information; do not disagree or argue.
You may have to repeat frequently.

NUTRITION: Patients with dementia may "forget" how to eat.
Check their dentures and check the temperatures of foods.
They may hide or hoard food; new foods may confuse them.
Eliminate distractions while eating, eliminate too many utensils, one will do.
They may be unable to decide what to eat, so serve one thing at a time.
They will need small pieces, and may "forget" how to chew.
This is called "Apraxia." You may need to remind them,
"You may chew now."

They may not be able to judge liquids; watch for choking.
Encourage fluids, they may "forget" how to drink.
This patient may need considerable help with feeding.
(This may present a problem in an acute care setting.)
Frequent finger foods may be better than regularly scheduled "meals."

ORIENTATION: Check their level of orientation frequently. It may alter dramatically during the day, and may even deteriorate considerably late in the day. (Sundowning) You may want to create large print calendars for them.

PERCEPTION: Due to the cognitive impairment, these persons may "see" things that are not there. They may also "hear" things unheard by others.
They may misinterpret data, such as curtains, reflections in windows or mirrors, etc.

QUERULENT: This person seeks reassurance and security. They may become complaining and fretful.
Avoiding answers heightens their insecurity.
Respond clearly and slowly and have them repeat what you said.
Use distraction techniques whenever necessary.
Avoid arguing, anger, rebuking.
Write down information if the patient can still read.

REPETITIOUS: This is vexing for caregivers. You will simply have to put on an extra dose of PATIENCE!!!

RESISTENCE TO INTERVENTIONS: This may happen because of fear or suspicion. Explain carefully and patiently.

SUNDOWNING: Agitated behaviors increase in the evening for some reason.
This may be due to a change in the level of light, or the person may be tired or stressed after a long day.
Further, YOU may be more tired and stressed after a long day....he WILL react to you.
Reduce the number of things going on at this time.
Reassure yourself the person is not doing this deliberately.
Plan for it.....prepare ahead of time for this problem!

SUSPICIOUSNESS: This patient may accuse you unreasonably, even of stealing or abuse. Be very careful.
This is usually due to the dementing process, but may also be due to a superimposed delirium from the illness or from medications.

STUBBORNNESS: A person who has always been stubborn may be worse now.
If he cannot remember when something happened, he may be "insulted" when told to do it.
Be certain your requests are understood.
Take the path of least difficulty; avoid arguments; accept compromise; don't take it personally!

TIME, SENSE OF: The patient who forgets quickly has no way to measure the passage of time.
Dementing diseases affect the internal clock.
This may affect sleeping, waking, and eating.
Medications may make it worse, especially at night.
This person may feel left alone for hours when you are out of sight for just a few minutes.

UNDERSTANDING: This person has difficulty comprehending what you say.
This is often misinterpreted as uncooperative behavior.
They will also quickly forget what was said.
They may say they understand when they do not from fear of embarrassment or reprisal.
They may have trouble understanding even written words; even when they can still read!
Reading and understanding are two different skills.
This person may not be able to make himself understood. He may not remember what something is called or may forget what he started to say.
Patience and creativity are required to help him to figure it out.
"That white thing" may be a blanket, a Kleenex, or a glass of milk....keep an open mind.

VISITORS: This person has agnosia, which means that they may not recognize people.
Avoid confusion; too many people at once.
This person may say that no one has come to visit when they just left.
When you visit a physician do not assume your patient will understand or remember the doctor's instructions.
Make notes, make yourself part of the process.

VERBAL AGGRESSION: This may be triggered by excessive environmental demands, frustration, fear, loneliness, loss, anxiety, helplessness.
Step back, think through what is happening.
Don't argue, contradict, or try to reason.
Sympathize, empathize, stay calm, speak softly.
Use distraction techniques or change the subject.

WEIGHT LOSS: This may happen suddenly in a strange environment.
Monitor eating carefully.
It is not good to plunk down a tray and walk away, leaving the person to fend for himself, then clean up later and say to yourself, "Well, he didn't eat again!"

WORRY: Who doesn't? This patient worries due to his dementing illness. Other family members may worry if the patient is telling them incorrect or conflicting information. Keep everyone informed and involved if at all possible.

X-FILES: You may feel you are dealing with an alien being!
This patient is certain he is in an alien world.
Think of how you might feel and how frightening it must be.

YOUR FEELINGS: Examine, correct, contain wherever it is necessary.
It is very important for YOU to remain in control!
Persons with cognitive impairments will react to even the smallest things.
This cannot be overstated!!
You cannot control his feelings, you CAN control your own.

ZYPREXA/ZOLOFT/OTHER DRUGS: These patients are often on "polypharmacy." That means many drugs, often from many physicians.
Drugs interact differently in the elderly, they will have to be managed carefully.
Often drugs are the cause of some of their problems.
Understanding is better than medicating.
Check with your primary physician and/or your local
Pharmacist often concerning medications.

Remember, even the smallest change of environment, routine, or caregiver can produce high stress in these patients, and these things are always present in the acute-care setting. These persons are unable to plan, initiate, or carry through voluntary activities. They may refuse to attempt any activity they cannot complete, such as washing, dressing, eating, or toileting. If it is at all possible, a known sitter should be provided when these patients are admitted to an acute care facility to provide a level of consistency. A change in environment may even extend to items left in the room that were not there before such as a stethoscope, a bedpan, a breathing treatment device…use your imagination. Similarly, overwhelming or competing stimuli are easily misinterpreted by such patients. In an acute care setting there is always high noise levels, multiple activities, and groups or crowds of strange people.

CHAPTER 9:

SELF-CARE FOR CAREGIVERS:

1)   . Learn stress reduction techniques and breathing techniques.
2)   Learn how and when to simply walk away from what you cannot handle.
3)   Take a CPR class.
4)   Purchase a cell-phone if you don't already have one, and keep it in your pocket at all times.
5)   Expect problems from family and friends who do not understand what you are going through. Explain what you can, forgive whatever they do, and continue to do your best for your loved one anyway.
6)   How to dress:
    Avoid necklaces, scarves, hoop earrings that may be grabbed or pulled.
    Wear your hair up, so it cannot be grabbed.
    Avoid other things or clothing items that could be grabbed.
    Wear comfortable clothing with plenty of pockets.
    Wear shoes that are comfortable and supportive, like tennis shoes.
    Learn how to keep a journal or do creative writing for yourself.

CAREGIVER'S BILL OF RIGHTS

Providing care for a person with Alzheimer's disease is often a stressful and demanding ordeal. It is important to remember that caregivers have human needs and emotions. They must care for the patient as well as themselves. The Alzheimer's Family Relief Program's "Caregiver's Bill of Rights" offers some tips for coping:

IT IS ALRIGHT TO:

BE ANGRY. Turn this energy into positive action. Clean closets, take a walk, talk with someone.

BE FRUSTRATED. Stop the present activity, take a deep breath and begin a different activity.

TAKE TIME ALONE. A favorite chair in a quiet room, a trip to the store or a few hours out with friends.

ASK FOR HELP. Explore family, friends and local agencies for resource services. Most doctors' offices and clergy can make referrals.

TRUST YOUR JUDGEMENT. Relax, you are doing the best you can.

RECOGNIZE YOUR LIMITS. You are a valuable person. Take care of yourself, too!

MAKE MISTAKES. No one is perfect. This is how we learn.

GRIEVE. This is a normal response to a loss. You may be sad over the loss of the way things used to be.

LAUGH AND LOVE. It may seem out of place, but your capacity to feel is not gone and can occur unexpectedly.

HOPE. Tomorrow, the day may go smoother, a friend may call, a cure may be found.

CHAPTER 10:

HOME SAFETY INFORMATION

The purpose of this chapter is to provide a quick and efficient response by persons in the household in the event of specific disasters. You will have enough other things on your mind – you don't need to be caught unaware in a disaster.

Disasters are natural or manmade events which cause major disruption in the environment of living such as damage to the building or grounds due to events such as severe wind storms, tornadoes, earthquakes. Also included are events that impact the activities of daily living such as loss of utilities (power, water, phone, television) due to an accident or an emergency within the house or in the surrounding community that disrupts the normal flow of activity.

I. SECURITY:

Crime Prevention:
Be cognizant of suspicious activity around the home or in the neighborhood.
Notification to law enforcement should be immediate if there is a crime in progress or in the event of extreme emergency or potentially life-threatening situation.
DO NOT give out any information over the telephone, except to the agency you have called, such as address, phone number, names of residents, or employment information.

IDENTIFICATION:
Create a written list of names of family and friends who are approved to visit in the home with your patient when you are not present.
Make it clear to sitters that no one else is approved for entry into the house unless prior arrangements have been made and you have been notified of such arrangements. For your own safety and protection as well as theirs this must include their own personal family and friends.

ENTRY ACCESS CONTROL:
Access to the house should be through the main front door and should be limited to the above identified family and friends or specially identified maintenance or repair persons who have made prior arrangements.

LIGHTS:
Adequate lighting should be available in all parking areas, walkways, entry and exit points.
Replace burned out bulbs immediately as needed.

TELEPHONES:
Most of what follows applies to sitters, however, it may also be useful to you as well:

Keep personal calls to a minimum and to no longer than five minutes in duration. Your patient can get into some real trouble very quickly when you are distracted.

Sitters should not move or delete any items from the Caller ID.

Keep a list of written messages as necessary in a notebook beside the telephone. If the caller is a solicitor, you can respond as follows:

"Thank you for calling, but we will not be interested." And hang up immediately.

An approved list of callers who may talk to your patient is the same as the list of approved visitors. Sitters should not encourage anyone else to talk to your patient. Take a message and promise a return call.

MAINTENANCE PROBLEMS/SAFETY HAZARDS:
First, a sitter should attempt to contact you. If unable to reach you or in an emergency use the following:
(Fill in the blanks for your own situation.)
Electric Company:
Power Outages:
Water/Sewer:
Gas Company:
Your Plumber:
Your Electrician:
Water turn-off location:
Electricity turn-off location:
Gas turn-off location:

II. INTERNAL DISASTER:

POWER FAILURE:
Check individual appliance/electric equipment to see if it is plugged into the wall. Check to see whether the cord is frayed or broken. If it presents a danger unplug it immediately.
Check the Electric Box (located:_____) to see whether one of the breaker switches has been thrown. Attempt to turn on the breaker. If it won't stay on, leave it off, and make a note, or call for help._____.
Check to see whether neighbors have electricity. If so, call your Power Company to inquire about the problem.

WATER PROBLEMS/FLOOD:
Turn off water if possible at the source (under the sink, behind the toilet, at the garden hose spigot, behind the water heater).
If this does not work, know the location of the main water meter. Open the water box and turn it off at the source from the street.
If this doesn't work, call your local utility company:_____.

FIRE:
KNOW what to do in case of a fire:
Where your extinguishers are located
How to use them: (P A S S)

Pull: break the seal and remove the pin
Aim: point nozzle at the base of the fire, 8-10 ft back from it.
Squeeze: the handle to emit chemicals
Sweep: from side to side beginning at the base of the fire.
Locations of all exits from the house (front door, back door, garage door, windows as necessary).
Evacuation procedures: Act calmly, DO NOT exhibit panic, move slowly and surely toward exits and remove all persons/animals from the house.

KNOW a safe procedure:
Rescue all persons/animals in the house as necessary first.
Alarm: (Call 911)
Contain the fire by closing doors wherever possible.
Extinguish the fire, when safe to do so, and evacuate as necessary.
Exit the house by the FRONT door if possible; if not, remember to take keys with you for locks on backyard gates and doors.
Go to a neighbor's house and call_____.

MEDICAL PROBLEMS:
For minor medical problems:
      Use the items in your First Aid Kit (You DO have one, don't you?)
      Use Advil for minor headaches
      Use Ice or Heat for minor pain or swelling
      Call _____at_____with any questions.

For major medical problems:
      Call 911 for major injury, heart attack, or stroke
      Immediately call _____
      Ensure that emergency personnel take a copy with them of:
            Health Care Directives
            Living Will
            Power of Attorney
            Health Care Surrogate
(Keep copies of these documents in a plastic Ziplock bag in a safe and convenient location – perhaps beside your telephone!)
      Think of your pets:
            Put dogs or cats outside or in their cages BEFORE emergency personnel arrive on the scene to keep them out of their way! Or at least put them in a room where you can shut the door to keep them contained.

III. EXTERNAL DISASTERS:

SEVERE THUNDERSTORMS:
Stay indoors, stay away from windows; do not use computers.
Do not use the telephones except for emergencies.
If the power goes out during the daytime – just wait for it to come back on.

If the power goes out after dark – use the flashlights you have positioned around the house in appropriate places.
Do not light candles, or attempt to light a fireplace in the dark.
Use battery powered radios to tune in to emergency stations for information.

TORNADOES:
A WATCH means one is likely to develop; stay tuned to TV or radio for further details. Use your weather radio if you have one.
A WARNING means one has actually been sited.
> GO IMMEDIATELY into a designated place.
> Take pillows and blankets and battery radio.
> Take your pets along with you.
> Stay there until the tornado passes and the all clear is given; or until rescue personnel arrive.

EARTHQUAKE:
Stay indoors; do not go outside to see what happened.
Get under a sturdy table, desk or interior doorway.
Stay away from fireplaces, windows, tall bookcases, and anything that could fall on you.
Turn on the radio and the TV for official announcements/information.
Turn off all electricity, water, gas if they are damaged or leaking.
Do not use the telephone unless it is an emergency.
Create an "Emergency Duffle-Bag" and know its location.

SEVERE WINTER STORM:
Monitor the TV and radio for information and announcements.
Gather blankets, warm clothing, emergency duffle-bag, flashlights.
Stay inside, keep the thermostat on a reasonable temperature and use more clothing and/or blankets to keep warm.

IV. HOUSEHOLD EQUIPMENT/UTILITIES MANAGEMENT:

HEAT/AIR CONDITIONER/THERMOSTAT:
The thermostat is located _____.
It is best to keep the heat setting at 68 degrees.
It is best to keep the air conditioner setting at 80 degrees.
You may turn the thermostat off if you feel too hot or too cold.
Wear more clothing, sweaters, blankets if you are cold.
Wear less clothing, open windows if you are hot.

WATER AND TURN-OFF VALVE:
There are usually turn-off valves under each sink, behind each toilet, and behind your water-heater. If necessary you can always turn off the main valve from the street to your home if you know the location.

TRASH:
Know which day your trash is collected and remember to have it ready.
Your patient may rummage in trash and get injured or sick.

VEHICLES:
Create a regular maintenance schedule for your vehicles. You will not want the added frustration of an unexpected breakdown.

INFORMATION FOR SITTERS:
Create a written list of instructions for any sitters.
Make certain that they are familiar with the symptoms of dementia and are patient and caring persons.
Make certain that they are familiar with all of the aforementioned information concerning safety and hazards in your home.

V. NECESSARY PHONE NUMBERS:

EMERGENCIES: 911
Fire Department (non-emergency)   _____

Police Department (non-emergency) _____

Local Poison Control Center   _____

NEIGHBORS:
To the left: _____   _____

To the right: _____   _____

Across the Street: _____   _____

Behind your house   _____   _____

FAMILY:
Children: _____   _____

                                   _____   _____

                                   _____   _____

OTHER: _____   _____

CHURCH: _____   _____

Where Did I Put My Map?

Pastor: _____ _____

Family Physician: _____ _____

<u>MISCELLANEOUS ITEMS:</u>
Keep a list of family members near your telephone:
    Be sure to include names, addresses, phone numbers, and relationship!

Keep a list of physicians, dentists, other health care providers;
    Include names, addresses, phone numbers, and HOURS they can be reached.

CHAPTER 11:

RECORD-KEEPING

Caring for your loved one with a dementing illness such as Alzheimer's Disease will take every ounce of effort you can muster up every minute of the day and night. Simplifying your life is not a luxury, it is a MUST! Now is the time to get things in order, you will be glad you did.

Create a list of your budget and your bill-paying information.
> You can use a ledger or a three-ring binder for convenience.
> Keep it up-to-date each month.

Keep copies of all necessary health care information in a Ziplock bag so it can easily be given to emergency medical personnel. Keep originals in a safe place.
> A Living Will
> Durable Power of Attorney
> Health Care Surrogate

Purchase a document file at your local office supply store so you can know where important documents are and that they are secure:
> Deed to your home
> Vehicle Titles
> Insurance Policies
> Wills, POA, Health Care Surrogate, Advance Directives
> Funeral Information
> Banking Information
>> Appoint a trusted person with a co-signature for emergencies.
>> Know what should be recorded at your court-house.

CREATE YOUR OWN RESOURCE LIST:

Alzheimer's Association
Hospice
Home Health Aids
Legal Information
Home Maintenance/Lawn Care
Insurance Companies
Vehicle/Transportation Information

Specialty Institutions
Family Services
Tax Information
Financial Consultants
Plumber/Electrician, etc.
Health Care Providers
Help with Paying Bills

CHAPTER 12:

A DAY IN THE LIFE OF H.B. GANN

January 2001

This is a true story of one day in the life of a person with Alzheimer's Disease. It is not embellished; it is not a medical treatise; it is just the straight-out truth about daily life.

It is very difficult to live with this disease. The physical body of someone you love is in front of you, but that person is no longer inside. There is no cure. There is no going back. The person you once knew is gone forever and some alien person is living in the body. It walks and talks; and although it occupies an adult body it is more like a newborn baby. It cannot always control its bodily functions. It wets its pants, or does its bowel movements in strange places. It drools and it kicks its feet and hits at you. It won't eat, or can't eat, but it unexpectedly demands more food. It calls you names it never even thought of before. It doesn't remember who you are, but it wants you to take care of it. Life as it used to be hangs suspended as you try to adjust to living with this alien being.

Anyone who has not personally lived it cannot truly understand what it is like to experience this "Long Goodbye." It is frustrating and tiring. It depletes every emotion you have. Caring for this person with Alzheimer"s Disease requires emotional strength and stamina, courage, and fortitude. Just when you think you have a handle on something, everything changes. In a very real sense, the caregiver, whoever that may be, is as much a victim of the disease as the person who has it. Not only does one experience shock, denial, fear, depression, and feelings of rage or helplessness, but financial considerations become a very real and very big problem. It is my hope that our story will help to bring some small understanding to the family of someone with this disease, or at least bring a better picture of the reality of daily life to folk who are not directly involved in caregiving. Those who are directly involved do not need someone to tell them what it is like.

This is also therapy for me. Family and friends tend to disappear when Alzheimer's enters the picture just when they are needed the most. What follows is ONE actual day:

4:00 a.m.: The day began earlier than I would have liked. I awoke when HB began to get restless in his sleep and I knew it meant he needed to use the bathroom. I laid still and waited until he woke up a little more to speak to him. When he opened his eyes I asked, "Would you like to get up and go to the bathroom?" He replied sleepily, "No, you go on without me if you want to, I've got to go to the bathroom before I wet my pants."

I got up and turned on the light in the hallway and returned to offer him my arm to help him stand up. He pushed my arm away and said, "Get out of my way, I know what I'm doing." I stepped back as he sat up on the side of the bed and tried to take off his pants. He could not get them off, of course, because he was sitting on them. He became very frustrated. I told him that it would work better if he could stand up and come into the bathroom with me. He stood up, opened the closet door, and began to pull down his pants in order to urinate in the closet.

I cried out, "Wait, wait, wait until we can get into the bathroom." I tried to convince him that the closet was not the toilet, but he just kept pushing me away. I suggested that he could follow me into the bathroom and that was the best place to do this. He wouldn't move. He had his underpants down to mid-thigh and had a tight grip on them. I reached for his arm to lead him out of the closet, and again he pushed my arm away hard and said, "Get out of my way, I know what I'm doing." I stepped back and said "Please don't pee in the closet, if you will just follow me I will show you where the bathroom is." He pushed me again and shouted, "I've got to go before I wet my pants, now leave me alone, I know what I'm doing." And proceeded to step back into the closet. I took a deep breath and said very softly, "If you will come with me, I will show you where the toilet is." He sighed deeply and replied, "O.K., I'll go with you, but first I need to pee," and tugged at his pants again. I took hold of his arm and said, "Boy, this sure is frustrating, I really don't know what to do." He looked at me very puzzled and said, "O.K., O.K., I'll go, but then you have to let me pee." I led him the six feet or so around the corner to the bathroom door.

As I turned on the light he looked in and said, "Just what do you want me to do for you in here?" I replied, trying not to let my exasperation show, "Just sit down on the toilet and everything will be O.K."

He stepped into the bathroom and opened the shower door. "That's not it, please just sit down here on the toilet," and I patted the seat of the toilet.

He studied the toilet for a moment, and shook his head. "I just can't do that," he said.

"Sure you can," I said, "all you have to do is turn around and sit down right here," again patting the toilet seat.

He looked into the shower again and said, "But those people in there (pointing into the shower) will steal everything we have and run away." I tried to reassure him, "Don't worry, I won't let them do that, Please sit down here now."
"No, I just can't do that."
"Please sit down here."
"But I need to pee!"
"O.K., Please sit down here."
"But I have to have something to sit on." (As he stood over the toilet.)
"It's right under you, please sit down."
"Let me think about it."
"Please sit down."
"I don't think it will fit."
"Please sit down."
"I'm going to have to go to the bathroom and pee."
"O.K., Please sit down here."
"First I'll need a towel."
"Please sit down."
"Where is my wallet?"
"It is in the bedroom on the dresser, please sit down here now and you can pee."
"Where are my pants?"
"You have them on, please pull them down and sit down here if you have to pee."
"I just cannot do this anymore, I'm going to have to sit down right here and pee!"
"Thank you, and thank You, God!"

This had only taken 20 minutes of pleading and explaining, but he did finally sit on the toilet. He peed, passed a little gas, and then just sat there.

"Are you done now?"

"Let me think about it."

I left him there and went to go let the dog out to do his thing while I went upstairs to the bathroom myself. I let the dog back in the house, turned off the kitchen lights, and returned to the bathroom where he was still sitting right where I left him, staring at the wall.

"Do you need some help?"

"I think those three guys in there (pointing to the shower) came right in here and stole my wallet."

"Your wallet is laying on the dresser in the bedroom. Come with me and I will show it to you. Would you like some help getting up?"

"No, I know what to do, now you get out of my way. I need to call the police and tell them what those guys did."

"O.K., I will help you, do you want some toilet paper?" I pulled off a piece and folded it just like he always did and handed it to him. He put it in his pocket.

"O.K., stand up and I will help you."

"O.K., I will." He pulled his pants further down and tried to take off his socks.

"You don't have to do that just now, just stand up and I will help you."

I reached for his pants to help pull them up, but he hit me in the face. I left the room and shut the door. I went back into the kitchen and sat down. (Just focus on breathing!)

Ten or fifteen minutes passed, it was now after 5:00 a.m. I was so tired; I leaned against the wall, closed my eyes, and said a little prayer, "Please, I need some help here, Lord!"

A voice in the bathroom said, "Now what did you want me to fix in here, I would just as soon go home and go to bed."

"That's a great idea, let's go!" I returned to the bathroom where he was still sitting without moving. I pulled his pants up to his knees.

"What are you doing?"

"Helping you get up, come on, now." He pounded on my back as I bent over, but I just kept on tugging at his pants, saying, "O.K., now you can stand up."

Suddenly, he stood up and I quickly pulled up his pants the rest of the way.

"O.K., Baby, now come with me." I motioned for him to follow me into the bedroom.

"Wait, I have to check something out first." He opened the shower door again. "I have to check in here."

"See, there is nothing in there."

"Boy, you sure are dumb. That is because those three guys that were in here took everything."

"Well, don't worry. I will take care of it, just come on with me and we will go back to bed."

He finally took a couple of steps toward the hallway, and I started to think, "This is just great." But I should have known that it was just too soon for that.

As we reached the door to the bedroom, he suddenly stopped, braced himself against the doorjamb, and refused to enter the room. "I don't want to go in there with all those people," he said.

I reached around him and turned on the lights in the bedroom. He looked surprised and said, "Well, look-a-here, they have a bed just like ours."

"It is ours, and you can just crawl in and lay down if you want to."

"You know, I think I will just do that, you don't think anyone will care do you?"

"No, that would be a great idea, just go ahead." He moved toward the bed and stood near the edge.

"Just go ahead and lay down now."

"I can't." (Just focus on breathing.)

"Sure you can, just sit down on the edge and lift up your legs and lay down. I picked up the covers and held them up for him to put his feet underneath them. He suddenly leaned back in the bed and kicked me hard with both feet. As he kept on kicking, I pulled up the covers over his legs and leaned over to kiss him to reassure him. As I leaned over he suddenly hit me in the face. (Just focus on breathing, just focus on breathing.)

I turned out the light and left the room, shutting the door behind me. It was now 6:30 a.m., I was exhausted, and all we had done was get to the bathroom. The day hadn't even started yet!

I went into the kitchen and poured a cup of coffee, I put it into the microwave to heat it while I fed the dog and the fish, and I went upstairs. I thought I might as well get dressed. I was up and awake and HB was back in bed. I brushed my teeth and my hair and put on my clothes.

As I came back down to the kitchen, I heard a noise in the bedroom. When I opened the door, there he stood. He had stripped the sheets off the bed; they were lying on the floor. He had put on two pair of pants over his pajamas.

He had six or eight shirts lying on the now bare mattress. The window shades were pulled up, the lights were on, all of his shoes were in a pile in the corner, and three rolls of toilet paper were in shreds in the bathroom. As I opened the door and gasped in surprise, he smiled broadly and said, "Well, look who's here, where are you living at now-a-days?"

He looked at me hopefully and said, "I guess I'm going to need some help to find Jude (me), I don't know where she has got to, and I can't find my pants."

Actually, I was not quite certain just where to begin. So I said, "I will just help you with this, Baby. Come over here and sit on the side of the bed. Thankfully, he let me help him take off the extra pants and the pajamas. I suggested that since he already had his clothes off, he might like to get into the shower where it was nice and warm, and get cleaned up before he started the day. He agreed, and I silently shouted "Hallelujah!" He followed me into the bathroom again and I turned on the water in the shower so it would be the right temperature before he stepped into it. He asked me whether "those guys" had left yet, and I reassured him there was no one there but the two of us. I handed him a washcloth and led him into the shower.

After he was safely inside and actually standing under the running water, I stepped outside the bathroom door, to remove my watch and my long-sleeved shirt I had on like a jacket. When I returned, he was still standing there right where I had left him. I told him I would help him; I reached for the bar of soap, and rubbed it on his tummy. He got very agitated, and said, "Get that stuff off of me right now!" He began flailing around trying to hit at me. I didn't want him to slip in the wet shower, so I stepped back and said, "O.K., I will take it off RIGHT NOW!"

I reached for the hand-held shower so I could rinse the soap off of his tummy, but he grabbed the shower away from me and proceeded to spray down the entire bathroom from ceiling to floor and me as well.

I reached over and turned off the water, handed him a towel, and walked out of the room. I shut the door behind me. (Just focus on breathing.) It is certainly one way to clean the bathroom, although it is definitely not my first choice.

I went upstairs and dried myself off and put on dry clothes. I returned to the bathroom and hesitantly opened the door. He was still in the shower with the towel, just standing there, doing nothing but holding the towel. I said, "Would like for me to help you?"

"I don't know what this thing is for." He said, referring to the towel.

"Well, come on out here and I will help you."

"I can't come out there because I am all wet."

"If you will step out here, I will help you get dry."

He finally stepped out of the shower and I encouraged him to follow me into the bedroom where there was more room, so I could dry him off and help him dress. He complied. We went into the bedroom and I began to use the towel to dry him off. He pushed me away, saying, "Don't put that thing on me. Now, I'm not going to tell you again."

"It is a towel, you can use it to dry yourself off. Here, I will give it to you and you can do it for yourself if you would like to."

I handed him the towel, he looked at it for a moment and said, "You are going to have to do it, I don't know how."

I finished drying him off and put on his underwear. He was using disposable paper briefs by now. We got them on without incident, as well as his undershirt, pants, and regular shirt. He sat on the edge of the bed for me to put his socks on and I hunched down to pull them on for him. He suddenly shouted, "DON"T YOU TOUCH MY FEET!" and kicked me in the face. My glasses went flying across the room, and I found myself on the floor. (Just focus on breathing.)

I stood up and offered him his slippers. He stepped into them as if nothing had happened. There was still a lot to do, but I was inspired by the thought that if we got finished he might go to his favorite chair and take a nap.

He followed me back into the bathroom and actually sat down on the closed toilet seat without complaint. I wet my hands and reached over to comb his hair. He slapped my hands away and shouted, "Don't you put that stuff on my hair!"

"It's O.K., it's just water, let me use the comb here and we will be done with it." I combed down his hair, while he complained the whole time that he didn't like "that stuff" put on his head, and I was just stupid because I just didn't understand that. But I just kept on combing, and we finally got it done.

Then I plugged in the electric razor. He pulled away from me, saying, "What are you going to do to me now?" I said, "This is your electric razor. Would you rather do this yourself?" I handed him the razor. He threw it across the room, shouting, "This thing is going to bite me, get it away."

I picked up the razor and ran it across my hand, saying, "See, it doesn't hurt me, would you like to try it?"

He took the razor and ran it across his hand like I had done. Then he handed it back to me and said, "You had better do this, I don't know how to do it." I shaved him as best I could. It is hard to do that to another person. I was afraid to push too hard for fear of "burning" him, but it didn't seem to be cutting like I thought it should. Maybe I just needed to buy a new inner part for it, I thought, I'd see about that later.

When I had finished shaving him, I put about a teaspoon of mouthwash into a small glass with some water to dilute it, and told him to use it to rinse out his mouth. He happily took the glass and proceeded to drink the mouthwash. I guess it couldn't hurt him, it was such a small amount; and anyway, at least it accomplished rinsing out his mouth. I washed his dentures and rinsed them and handed them to him to put back into his mouth. He pulled away from me again, saying, "Now, don't do that. Only a dentist can do that."

"We don't need a dentist, you can just put these teeth back into your mouth like you always do yourself."

"You don't understand. They have to be fixed just right. Only a dentist can do it. Anyway, I already have some and I don't need these."

"Look into the mirror, your mouth is empty. These are your very own teeth, made just to fit into your mouth, and they will fit in very easily if you just slip them in."

"Well, O.K., I will use these temporarily, but someone else is going to be looking for them and I will be out some teeth." He finally placed the dentures in his mouth and smiled at himself in the mirror.

It was now 8:30 a.m., and it had already been a long day. He followed me into the kitchen and I showed him where to sit down at the table while I fixed him some breakfast.

I went to the cupboard and got out his pills and a glass of water. I handed him the first pill, which was a rather large pink pill, and he put it in his mouth and started to chew it like candy, making a face.

I said, "No, No, you don't have to do that. Just swallow it down with the water." So he drank the whole glass of water down, but still had the pill in his mouth. I got him to spit it out into my hand and I took it back into the kitchen and crushed it in the pill-crusher. I put the crushed pill into a spoonful of Orange Sherbet Ice Cream, mixed it well, and took it back to him. He didn't want to take it, but I told him it was Ice Cream, so eventually he took it in his mouth. I thought he was going to swallow it, and I leaned over closer to him to watch. He spit it out into my face.

So much for that one, I thought. I gave him his liquid vitamins in a little medicine cup, expecting him to spit that out as well. He happily swallowed it down, saying, "That stuff is really good! I wouldn't mind having some more of that." I told him that had been all he needed for now.

I cut up a banana and a banana-walnut muffin into bite-sized pieces, poured a can of vanilla Ensure into a glass, and offered them to him. He thanked me, but just sat there looking at it. I sat down beside him and began to eat my muffin, thinking it would give him the right idea of what to do with the food. He still sat there. I picked up a piece of the muffin and offered it to him, saying, "This is your favorite banana-walnut muffin, and you can eat it now." He pushed my hand away, and said, "I'm too full to eat right now. Don't you remember, I just got through eating that whole big plate full of hamburgers and french-fries, and I don't have room for this stuff now. Maybe later." He got up from the table and went into the family room toward his chair.

I was frustrated and disappointed, but I followed him into the other room and helped him sit in his chair. I put the glass of Ensure on the table beside his chair and turned to walk away. He picked it up and drank it down completely. Then he said, "This sure would have been good if only I had some breakfast to go with it."

I shook my head and went back into the kitchen to get his breakfast I had prepared. I put all the pieces into a plastic soup bowl, got a spoon, and took it to him. He shoveled it down like he was starving as he glanced around from time to time to see if I was watching. When he had finished eating he stood up and said,

"If you will show me the bathroom, I have to drain my lizard." My heart sank, but I said, "Come with me, I'll show you where it is."

This time when we reached the bathroom, he actually went in by himself and used the toilet without any problem. When he came back out he returned to his chair. He said, "I am just exhausted from having to tell those guys again and again where to put that steel. They never listen, and if they aren't careful management is going to see what they are doing and they will lose their jobs. I am sure glad that I am not in their shoes." He sat down, leaned back, and closed his eyes. I thought, "Good, he is going to take a nap, so I will go in and clean up the bathroom and the bedroom." As soon as he started snoring I headed for the bathroom. I had no more than picked up a towel than I looked behind me and there he stood. He said, "I've got to find my car keys because I am going to cut down those trees out front today and I need to go get my saw."

I walked him back to the family room and said, "You can do that later, why don't you just sit down here and rest for a while."

36

"You know, that's a great idea, I haven't done anything but work, work, work today and I am ready for a nap." Again, he sat down in his recliner.

I turned on the TV and found something I thought he would like to watch and returned to the bathroom. I hurried to get it cleaned up and took the towels upstairs to the laundry room. When I came back downstairs he was standing at the front door looking outside. I asked, "What are you looking for?"

"Well, Jude left, and I don't know where she went. I don't like to be in this place alone, I want to go home."

"I am Jude, I haven't gone anywhere, and this is our home. You can just be here anywhere you want to be and it's O.K."

"Are you sure those people won't mind if we stay here? I kind of like this place, it is really nice, and I wouldn't mind if we stayed here."

"I am very certain, this is really our own house. Come on back here with me and we will find us a place to sit down and watch TV."

I herded him back into the family room again, and sat him down in his recliner. I sat down on the couch, hoping that would encourage him to stay put. Not for long. He got up and wandered around the room, looking at the bookshelves and the magazines, and the pictures of family sitting around here and there. I steeled myself to sit still and let him wander and look. He picked up an end table, the magazines on its lower shelf spilled out onto the floor. I jumped up and went over to where he was standing. I was afraid that he would slip on the magazines and fall. I said, "Here, let me help you with that. What did you want to do with it?"

"Well, I have told you all that I'm going to that this pile of steel needs to be put over there. If you won't cooperate I will just have to file a complaint against you and I promise you that you won't like that one little bit. If you have never had a complaint filed I'm the one to tell you how to do it and do it right."

"Let's put this down right here and move away from here so no one slips and falls down. Then you can come on around here and make yourself comfortable in this chair while I clean up this 'pile of steel.'"

"It's about time you decided to do as I tell you." He skirted the spilled magazines and headed for the back door. "I'm going back here to the warehouse and check on that furniture that those guys delivered today, I'll be right back."

I just let him go because the back yard is fenced in and locked up, and I knew he wouldn't stay outside very long because the temperature was 20 degrees. He stepped out the door, looked around for a few minutes, and came back inside.

"I'll tell you what," he said, "it is just too cold for me to want to work out there today."

"Good thinking, why don't you come sit over here and I will get you something to read."

As he took the magazine I handed him and sat down again, I glanced at the clock. It was 11:30, I couldn't believe where the morning had gone. It was almost time to have lunch. I really did not want to even deal with that; but I began to think through what I could put together to eat that could be cut up into small bites.

He doesn't always know how to use spoons, forks, and knives anymore. I thought back of any recipes I knew that would serve my purpose, and then I remembered that I had a couple of hotdogs. I told him to just relax and read his magazine while I fixed us something to eat for lunch. I microwaved a couple of eggs, popped in some toaster hashbrowns, cut up the hotdogs and a piece of cantaloupe I still had, and opened a small bottle of orange juice. I put everything on our plates, put them on the table, and called him into the kitchen to eat. He sat down and I tied his towel-apron I had made around his neck and pushed him up to the table.

He sat very still, looking at the food, not saying anything for a moment. Then he stood up, pulled off his apron, and said, "I don't have time for this right now, I'm going to have to go out and mow the grass."

I said, "It's time to eat your lunch right now, we can go out and mow the grass after we finish eating." (There was snow on the ground.) He said, "Now, what did I tell you? I don't want this stuff right now. You are the stupidest person I have ever met." He picked up his plate and dumped it on the floor. "Now don't bother me with your petty little problems, I have important things to do." He went back into the family room and wandered around like he was lost. I asked him what he was looking for. He said, "Well, if you will show me where the bathroom is, I have to drain my lizard." (Just focus on breathing.)

I took him by the hand and led him back toward the bathroom. He followed slowly and hesitantly and finally asked, "Where are you taking me?"

"You said you needed to use the bathroom."

"Oh, you want me to clean your vacuum?"

"No, not now, do you need to pee again?"

"Well, I don't care, if you want to I guess we can."

"Then come in here and pull down your pants."

"Now why would I want to do that?"

"Because you said you needed to pee."

"Well, of course I do, I do it all the time. Here, just let me go get the vacuum."

"We don't need the vacuum right now, would you still like to drain your lizard?"

"I can't do that in here, I need to go find the bathroom. Now just step back and let me go before I wet my pants."

I tugged on his pants and told him he would need to just pull them down a little way and turn around and he would see that the toilet was right there waiting for him. I gently took him by the shoulders and tried to get him to turn around. He would not turn, but he did pull down his pants and leaned forward as if to sit down on the toilet seat.

I offered my arm to help him sit down but he just leaned forward a little more and proceeded to pee on the floor. Of course, it ran down his leg into his pants, his socks, and his shoes. I leaned against the bathroom door and took a deep breath. "Let me help you step out of your wet clothing, and we will find you something clean and dry."

After I had cleaned both him and the bathroom again, I decided that a ride in the car might be a good thing. He loves to ride and I needed to drive down to Franklin and check on our house down there anyway. I got his jacket out of the closet and held it up for him. I said, "Let's just take a little ride to Franklin, would you like that?"

"You need to go to work?"

"No, I don't work anymore. We can just ride down and check on our house in Franklin."

"Now, don't try to put that thing on me," he said, referring to the jacket, "It doesn't match my uniform or my shoes." I put it on him anyway.

He drug his feet and resisted walking out the garage door, but when he saw the car, he said, "I'll tell you what let's do, let's just go for a ride and try to calm down."

"Good idea, come and sit over here." I held the car door open for him. He struggled with figuring out just how to get into the car and I let him take his time. He finally got in and sat down and I reached across him and fastened the seat belt. I walked around the car and got in the driver's side. He said, "Now where are we going?"

We drove the 25 miles to Franklin without much difficulty. He talked the whole way about wanting to see if we could find his father because he had not called or visited and he was certain that he knew we had moved back to Kentucky. His father had passed away over twenty years ago, but I let him talk and promised that we would try to find him. When we arrived at our house I let him get out of the car and walk around with me as I checked everything out. He observed that it was a really nice house and he wouldn't even mind living there. He wondered if the people who owned it would consider selling it to us. He picked up a few leaves that were lying on the ground and put them in his pocket. I asked him why he wanted them. He replied in a whisper, "These things are very valuable and everyone would just come here and get them if they knew about them. Don't talk so loud, they will come and try to steal them away from me."

Things appeared to be in good shape, so I helped him get back into the car and we started back home. A few blocks out of town he said, "You are going the wrong way. I want to go home now." I reassured him that I knew where I was going and that we were headed in the right direction and that we would be home in a few minutes. He persisted, and wanted me to pull over and find a "State Policeman" so he could ask for directions home. I assured him that I was going the right direction as fast as I could and if he would sit back and relax we would be home in a few minutes. He fumbled with the seat belt for a few seconds and suddenly took it off. I said, "You need to keep that on because we are driving and it will keep you safe." He said, "I have told you for the last time that I want to go home now." I said, "I'm driving there as fast as I can, please relax and sit back." He sat quietly for a moment and suddenly he said, "Well, Okay, if you won't do what I tell you to I will just have to do it for myself!" He opened the car door and started to get out.

I grabbed him by the pantleg and held on for dear life while I slowed the car and pulled over to the side. He pulled against me and kept trying to get out. I begged him to trust me, and get back into the car. He finally sat back, and I started driving again. I kept my tight grip on his pants, and kept begging him to just sit still and relax.

I just kept driving; I wanted to get home as fast as possible. I held my tight grip on him as he continued to try to pry my fingers loose. I cried! I tried to focus on breathing, but I was really panic-stricken.

I said, "Please, please do not do this. I promise we are going home and we will be there shortly. And I promise that I will never take you this far away from home again." He just kept saying that I was a liar, and that if we ever did get home, he was going to just knock my head right off my shoulders for not doing what he wanted me to do. I told him that would be okay if he would just not open the car door anymore. As we finally turned the corner at our house he looked up and exclaimed, "Well, look-a-here, there's a house that looks exactly like ours!"

"It is our house, just like I said it would be."

"Well, for once I guess you were right. I am so tired from all that work we did I would just love to find me a place to sit down and take a nap."

"Thank you, Lord!" Later, a friend told me that the back seat of our car has "child-proof locks." I didn't even know that. Now whenever we go anywhere HB rides in the back seat, even though we never go that far from home anymore. I wish I had known that sooner, we could have both been killed. I am enormously grateful for the very capable Guardian Angel that God has assigned to us!

As we walked into the family room toward his favorite chair, I realized that it was only a little after 3:00, and the worst part of the day was yet to come.

Persons with Alzheimer's Disease experience what is called "sundowning." For some unknown reason, late in the afternoon as the sun begins to fade, their symptoms tend to get worse. For HB this usually occurred between about 4:00 p.m. and bedtime. I wished for some company to stop by and entertain him for a while, but no such luck.

He did sit in his chair and take a nap for about 20 minutes. When he woke up, of course, he needed to find the bathroom again. I felt like I was on a Merry-go-round from someone's nightmare and couldn't get off. After we went through a similar routine of finding the bathroom, figuring out why we were in there, refusing to sit down, and peeing on the floor again, I cleaned him up with dry clothes, washed the bathroom floor, let him back to his chair and collapsed on the couch.

HB sat down in his favorite recliner and I turned on the TV. After a few minutes he dozed off and began to snore. I was very grateful, and when the phone rang I grabbed it quickly so it would not awaken him. It was a friend of mine who called to chat. I had been sitting on the sofa with the cordless phone nearby. Since he was still sitting comfortably in the recliner and was still snoring, I stood up and walked toward the kitchen as I was talking on the phone. I took about two steps into the kitchen and turned around. There he stood, and he was holding the fishbowl. My heart sank. I didn't know exactly what to do.

"What do you want me to do with this?"

"Just let me have it, please."

"No, I can put it wherever you want it," as he pulled it back the water sloshed. I wondered if the little Beta fish in the bowl had any idea of what was about to happen to him.

"Please let me hold it for you and I will put it where it should go." My friend on the phone was laughing; I was preparing to catch the fishbowl when he dropped it.

I wondered whether to run for a towel or to just stand by until he handed me the fishbowl.

"I knew you would like this and these are really going to be a good selling item." He beamed. "We should order several to keep on hand, we can make a killing with these."

"Great idea, let's put this one down here on the coffee-table, O.K.?" He finally relinquished the fishbowl and I placed it back in its spot on the table. I told my friend that my "conversation time" was over and I would call her back another time.

HB headed for the kitchen saying, "I'm going to make something to eat. Would you want me to fix you something?"

"I will fix you anything you want, just tell me what you would like to have. But, please let me do the fixing."

"I believe I would like some popcorn."

"O.K., you go sit down in your recliner and I will bring it to you when it is ready."

He went down the hallway toward the garage door saying that he had to check to make sure everything was locked up back there. I put a package of popcorn in the microwave and kept an eye on him as he wandered through the house checking every door (even the closets and cupboards) to see whether they were locked.

He walked up and down the hallway several times, looking in each room and looking in each mirror very carefully. He peeked around the corner into the kitchen to see what I was doing, and then he surreptitiously tiptoed over to the hall closet and got out his coat. He started into the bathroom with the coat and tried to stuff it into the cupboard under the bathroom sink. I asked him if he needed some help to hang his coat back in the closet.

He whispered, "Don't let those guys hear you, shhhh."

"There are no 'guys' in here, only you and me."

"Shhhh, now don't talk too loud, they will hear you."

"Please let me hang up your coat."

"No," he kept on whispering, "I'm going to put it in here so they can't see it. Then I will have it whenever I am ready to use it and they can't take it away from me."

I let him put the coat under the sink. It seemed to make him happy. I led him into the family room and went to get his bowl of popcorn and a drink. He sat down and held the bowl in his lap doing nothing. I reminded him that he would have to eat the popcorn.

"Here, do you want to have this?"

"No, thank you, I have my own bowl."

"I am too full to eat this, you can have it if you want it."

"Why don't you just eat whatever you want of it and I will eat the rest." He took a couple of bites and put the bowl of popcorn on the floor for the dog.

I grabbed it up before the dog could get to it and set it on the coffee table. He drank his orange juice and closed his eyes to take a nap.

I had not taken two bites myself when he sat upright and said (of course), "Let's see now, does this house have somewhere people can use the restroom?"

"Yes, it does." I said. "Why don't you just come with me and after you use the restroom you can go to bed if you would like to."

"It would be really great if we could find a bed where I could lay down for a while, I just can't keep my eyes open."

We headed for the bathroom again and I prayed that we could actually get it done. We walked through the kitchen and into the back hallway. He peered around the corner cautiously. I assured him that we were headed toward the bathroom, and I reached in and turned on the light.

He walked on past me and peered into the bedroom saying, "There is too many people in there, I don't want to go in there."

I turned on the bedroom light. "See, no one here, only your bed. Would you like to get in it?"

"Yes, but I have to pee first."

"Would you like to go into the bathroom and try to use the toilet?"

"I will if there is no one else already in there."

I assured him that the bathroom was empty, and offered him my hand to lead him back down the short hallway into the bathroom. We entered the room and he went immediately to the shower doors. He opened them and looked in.

"Well, they are not in here."

"That's good, now you can use the toilet."

"What's wrong with it?"

"Nothing is wrong with it, just pull down your pants and go ahead and use it." I reached for his pants to help him. Bad idea! He slapped my hands away and said, "What are you doing?"

"Let's finish using the bathroom and get ready for bed. I will go get your pills while you use the toilet."

He followed me out of the bathroom and into the kitchen. I got his pill out of the cupboard and handed it to him with a glass of water. He pushed it away. He said he had already had some and I could have this one if I wanted it. I tried to encourage him to swallow the pill, but he wasn't interested right now. I suggested that we could just go to bed for now.

We went back into the bedroom and I helped him get undressed. I took off his glasses, he said, "Now, don't ever do that again or I will have to hit you." I took out his hearing aid, he said, "Now, I told you to leave my ears alone." I started to pull his shirt up over his head, he said, "Why are you doing this to me?" I said, "We need to take these things off before you can get into the bed." He let me pull the shirt over his head, but he wouldn't pull his arms out of the sleeves. After several minutes of trying and explaining, I finally got the shirt off. I thought about just letting him sleep in his clothes. It probably would have been the smart thing to do, but I persisted and asked him to stand up so we could remove his pants. He stood up and I thought he was going to cooperate with removing his pants. Wrong! He pulled down his pants, turned around toward the bed, and peed on the bed.

I took off his pants and shoes and got his pajamas, stripped the bed and put on clean linens. He sat down on the edge of the bed as if to lay down, and, of course, I leaned over to help him lift up his legs onto the bed. He leaned back and kicked me hard with both feet. I picked myself up off the floor, gathered the wet linens, and leaned over to kiss him goodnight. He said sweetly, "Goodnight, Darlin'" as if everything was just peachy.

I turned off the lights, shut the door, and headed toward the laundry room wondering just how long he would actually stay in the bed. After I put the linens in the washing machine and came back downstairs I peeked in to see if he was asleep. He was laying flat on his back in the bed, eyes wide open, slowly pulling the covers into a little ball on his belly. I decided to just leave him alone and let him try to go to sleep. In just a few minutes he was snoring.

I sat down on the sofa and thought about the events of this day. This was actually not a bad day. We have had worse; we have had better. I am learning to focus on breathing, this is a good thing. I am trying to be grateful for this precious gift the Lord has given to me. I know that "All things work for the good for those who love the Lord and are called according to His purpose." It's just that the mysterious ways of the Lord sometimes overwhelm me. HB is not suffering. He is in a place of special and tender care by the Lord. He seems to be happy most of the time even though he doesn't know where he is or who he is with. I guess you couldn't ask for much more than that in this life.

THE AUTHOR OF LIFE

When the Author of Life puts pen to the page

A new life on earth is begun,

And the chapters unfold as the story is told

Of the sorrows and joys in each one.

'Til at last, when the Author has finished His tale

and the last drop of ink is depleted,

It tells as it should, He pronounces it good,

And closes the book He completed.

Jude Gann
2001

CHAPTER 13:

CONNECTIONS AND RESOURCES

ALZHEIMER'S ASSOCIATION
919 North Michigan, Suite 1000
Chicago, Illinois 60611-1676
(800) 272-1900

ALZHEIMER'S DISEASE EDUCATION & REFERRAL CENTER (ADEAR)
P.O. Box 8250
Silver Spring, Maryland 20907-8250
(800) 438-4380

The 36 Hour Day (Revised Edition) 1991
       Mace, Rabins
       Johns Hopkins University Press
       Baltimore, MD

The Best Friends Approach to Alzheimer Care, 1997
       Bell, Troxel
       Health Professions Press
       Baltimore, London, Toronto, Sydney

Your local bookstore has many excellent books available on Alzheimer's Disease and on caregiving.

There are also many Web sites available on the Internet if you have access to a computer.

I have tried to share information and knowledge gleaned from the years of caring for my husband with Alzheimer's Disease.
This is not meant to be an exhaustive study of the disease, nor is it intended to be a detailed treatise on caregiving. If you want further information there is much to be found.

I hope you have found this little quick reference book to be useful, and I pray for the soon discovery of a cure for this disease.   -Your friend, Jude.

MEDICATION ADMINISTRATION RECORD

Medication	Dosage	Date/ Time	Date/ Time	Date/ Time	Date/ Time	Date/ Time	Date/ Time	Date/ Time	Notes:
MultiVitamin	1 tablet daily at 9am	---*E*	*X*	*A*	*M*	*P*	*L*	*E*	---

DAILY PROGRESS REPORT

ASSESSMENTS						INTERVENTIONS								NOTES
Date	Time	Temp	In (cc's)	Out (cc's)	BM s/ m/l	Bath	Shave	Teeth/ Dent's	Hair	Diaper change	Linens	Meds	Meal S/ M/L	

This form can easily be modified to fit your needs. It is, however, important to keep an accurate record of these items, both for your own information and for your physician.

MEDICAL INFORMATION

Place Photograph Here

NAME _____

ADDRESS _____
_____

PHONE( ) _____

Age _____ Sex _____ Race _____

Height _____ Weight _____

Blood Type _____ Code Status _____

Emergency Contact: _____

Phone: ( ) _____

Primary Physician: _____

Phone: ( ) _____

Health Insurance Numbers: _____

Policy # _____

Group # _____

MEDICATION ALLERGIES: _____
_____

Food/Other Allergies: _____
_____

Major Illness/Condition: _____
_____

Education Level: _____
_____

IMMUNIZATIONS:

Type: Month/Year

PPD _____

Flu Shot _____

Pneumonia Vaccine _____

Tetanus Booster _____

Hepatitis B _____

Rubella _____

RPR _____

Mumps/Rubeola _____

Other _____
_____

Chest x-ray _____

EKG _____

PSA _____

Pap Smear _____

Mammogram _____

Physical Exam _____

Dental Exam _____

Dentist: _____

Phone: _____

Eye Exam: _____

Phone: _____

Eye Doctor: _____

Phone: _____

MISCELLANEOUS NOTES:

HOME MEDICATIONS:

Pharmacy: _____

Phone: _____

Drug: _____ Strength: _____ When taken: _____

_____

_____

_____

_____

_____

Over-the-counter/Herbal Remedies:

_____

_____

_____

_____

Other Special Treatments (Specify):

_____

_____

_____

_____

_____

_____

_____

_____

MEDICAL HISTORY:

Cancer_____ Transplant_____
Transfusion_____ Reaction_____
Bone Problems_____ Arthritis_____
Falls_____ Artificial Limbs_____
Replacements (Circle) Hip   Knee
Shoulder Other_____
COPD_____ Tuberculosis_____
Asthma_____ Bronchitis_____
Allergies (specify)_____

Glasses_____ Contacts_____
Glaucoma_____ Cataracts_____
Hearing Deficit_____ Hearing Aid_____
Uses Sign Language_____
Dental Problems_____ Dentures_____
Speech Problems_____ Mute_____
Swallow/Chew Problems_____
Hepatitis_____ Jaundice_____
Anemia_____ Reflux_____
Ulcer_____ Shunts_____
Incontinent: Bowel_____ Bladder_____
Kidney Problems_____ Prostate_____
Diabetes_____ Accuchecks_____
Thyroid_____ Skin_____
Dialysis_____ Frequency_____
Heart Attack_____ Angina_____
CHF_____ Murmur_____
Palpitations_____ Arrhythmias_____
Hypertension_____ Hypotension_____

Seizures_____ Alzheimer's_____
Parkinson's_____ Stroke_____
Dementia_____ Confusion_____
Mental Illness_____ Other (Specify)_____

Tobacco Use_____ Alcohol_____
Drug Addiction_____ Type_____
Substance Abuse_____
Special Diet (Specify)_____
Fluid Restriction_____
Last Menstrual Period_____
Activity Restrictions (specify)_____

Food Preferences_____

Precautions: HIV/AIDS_____ Radioactive_____
Living Will_____ Location_____
Advance Directive_____ Location_____
POA (Name)_____
   Phone:_____
AT HOME THIS PATIENT USES:
Oxygen_____ Walker_____
Wheelchair_____ Hospital Bed_____
Hospice_____ Home Health_____
Other_____

Other important information:

_____

_____

SPECIAL NOTES:

www.ingramcontent.com/pod-product-compliance
Lightning Source LLC
Chambersburg PA
CBHW080443290526
45791CB00008BA/2594